Tears
A Key to a Remedy

PETER P. VAN OOSTERUM

Tears
A Key to a Remedy

ASHGROVE PRESS, BATH

Published by Ashgrove Press Limited
Bath Road, Norton St Philip, Bath BA3 6LW, UK

Distributed in the USA by
Words Distributing Company
7900 Edgewater Drive, Oakland,
CA 94621, USA

First published in English 1997

Originally published in Dutch as
Laat je tranen de vrije loop
©Uitgeverij Ankh-Hermes bv 1995

ISBN 1-85398-103-6

Typeset in 12/13¾ pt Caslon by
Ann Buchan (Typesetters), Shepperton
Printed in Great Britain by Redwood Books
Trowbridge, Wiltshire

CONTENTS

Preface   7
About the Instruments we call our Mind   9

CHAPTER ONE   The Organisation Man   13
CHAPTER TWO   Excretion   23
CHAPTER THREE   Body's Own Preparation Therapy   31
CHAPTER FOUR   Tears   41
CHAPTER FIVE   The Method   55

A Short Explanation of Tear Therapy   69

CHAPTER SIX   Diagnosis Using the Bio-tensor   71
CHAPTER SEVEN   A Few Case Histories   81
CHAPTER EIGHT   Conclusion   91

PREFACE

Over the past 30 years I have been involved in all kinds of natural health care. During these years we have seen an enormous shift in opinion towards these natural systems. In our part of the world this opinion shift has been something of a revolution.

During the sixties, when I first became interested in medicine, orthodox medicine did not consider natural systems worth bothering about. Any theory that arose from outside the university environment was considered questionable. In fact doctors told their patients that natural health practitioners were dangerous charlatans and many of my colleagues in those days were persecuted.

Nowadays, an increasing number of doctors are taking natural health care seriously. We now have organisations for doctors practising homeopathy, ortho-molecular health care, bio-resonance, herbal medicines, etc. The pharmaceutical industry has also taken up the challenge, and indeed the opportunity, and now supplies numerous natural health preparations and products

In its turn, natural health care has had to do a great deal of catching-up as far as thorough scientific research is concerned, in order to earn the trust of orthodox medical science.

A lot has been achieved, though some of the research and test methods used by medical science do not work for us. You cannot always repeat a natural process, and science demands tests that are repeatable at will. Yet natural health care systems have to be proven effective; and of course we all do like to prove things beyond the shadow of a doubt.

In the past the method used by natural health practitioners

was to produce case histories and statistical evidence. However, since the pharmaceutical industry has become involved, we are pleased to be able to say that our scientific credentials have improved.

I have written this book for professional colleagues as well as for lay people, in order to share a method which I have developed myself. Since the subject does not really lend itself to industrial research, I have used case histories to make and illustrate my point.

The degree of proof is increased by good case histories. I invite everybody who, after reading this book, starts working with this method, to send me their histories. Quite apart from that, every method is subject to improvements in efficiency. What we need is a growing body of experience fed by as much reaction from those who have used the method as possible.

In order to make this book accessible to all I have omitted medical jargon wherever possible. I am absolutely convinced that this method can never do harm.

This book is about a simple and inexpensive therapy that can be used to treat many emotional problems, as well as physical symptoms that may have an emotional basis. The basic material used in the method is tears, the clear fluid that drips down your cheeks when you are in an emotional state of mind.

Of course tears are not used in their natural form. They have to be processed into the right preparation in order to become an effective remedy.

The technique for this preparation is simple and easy for the non-professional to learn. This simplicity is another reason why I have tried to make this book as straightforward as possible.

I hope that many people will discover how much tension can be relieved and peace of mind and physical health restored using this simple method

Peter P. van Oosterum

About the instruments we call our mind; and about the potential to become and stay healthy and in harmony by using what we know about these instruments

Tears heal the mind

Shedding tears, crying, is something that our society has never looked upon with much esteem. Generally, people who cry are considered less well-balanced than they ought to be. They may be thought weak or unstable.

There *are* occasions when crying is admissible, for instance at the funeral of a loved one. However, on these occasions it is customary to wish strength and firmness to those in mourning and advise them to straighten up and look forward instead of back, because 'life goes on'.

Speaking in this way to a grieving person implies that we consider that life is only going well when no emotional storm or disturbance causes us to cry out or behave ourselves in any way guided by our inner sadness.

I consider that in this case society's reaction is undoubtedly peculiar and probably absurd. My aim here is to show how harmful this attitude is and how there is a better way for us to deal with it.

Subsequently, I hope to share with you a very simple, inexpensive method of making a sovereign remedy for yourself and others, out of tears. My aim is to supply you with a tool which is beneficial to people's mental health and stability.

For you to gain from this method there is only one real

precondition: you must be willing and able, if necessary on your own, to admit that in your mind and memory there are sad and painful things. I mean in particular those things whose impression lasted so much longer than the time they took to occur, thus causing you grief. You may not find this easy; but just consider that without these emotions you would not be human, you would be a machine.

There is unlikely to be anyone who has not covered up an old and painful wound somewhere in the cave of his or her memories. It is not really important what it is. The important thing is that old wounds that still hurt when touched are, to a greater or lesser extent, damaging to our ongoing lives. If we find that we are sometimes hurt by unbidden memories, this is a lead to follow.

If my findings are true, and I have many reasons to suppose that they are, then it really is time to make this knowledge and these simple techniques accessible to as many people as I can reach.

Our society suffers from many of the so-called diseases of civilisation. Quite a lot of these ailments are related to the way we handle our own and other people's emotions. Far too many people judge themselves solely according to their usefulness in life and to what other people think of them.

Vulnerability and weakness are not popular. Many people put themselves under stress in their attempts to conceal what they perceive as negative qualities. In effect they are using a form of mental violence against themselves which may hurt them more than any form of violence inflicted by anyone else. The violence we inflict on ourselves seems inevitable and justified to us. For this reason it probably the most traumatising form of violence there is.

The consequences, the permanent damage of this subtle self-torture can form self-reproducing traces throughout our organism. The coming-about of these chains we ourselves call 'learning', 'experiencing' and also 'suffering', but fortunately also 'enjoying'. It takes place throughout our body and, in the process, small protein-like molecules are used. These we produce ourselves; they are called neuro-transmitters. With them we programme the paths in our mental functioning and, through that, the consequences.

In most of the cases, when dealing with old, or recent grief, or with negative experiences which do not seem to make any sense to us, we are dealing with these chains of traces. They do not only direct us, they also keep us, quite literally, chained.

So many people have suffered severe loss in their lives, or have been submitted to violence or grief or torturing pain for long periods of their lives. And it will almost certainly not work if we tell such people that all their suffering is over and that there is no point in crying about it any more. These remarks certainly won't help anyone whose whole heart is still aching from what has happened.

This book is dedicated to a kind but effective way to release ourselves from chains from the past that too often keep us tied down in agony.

CHAPTER ONE

The 'Organisation' Man

We are all like a large, complex company with a board of directors, daily systems and routines, a continuously updated profit and loss account and a manufacturing plant working round the clock to produce a single product: the joy of life!

Some people give this product the name of one of the most important types of semi-finished goods: 'success'. But this will not do, for when success is not transformed into the joy of life through the use of all the tools available to the mind and body, comparable to internal testing, proving and certificating procedures, it will soon disintegrate into waste products such a boredom, idleness, uselessness and loss of interest which, in the end, will lead to disappointment.

We often see these malfunctions striking people who have chosen the earning of big money and success in business as their highest, indeed their only goal.

These people usually name the company, as we all do, by the small but highly significant word 'I'. This company manufactures a surplus of success which, therefore, no longer has special meaning in the eyes of the boss. Subsequently, success is squandered and the production of the main product, the joy of life, loses efficiency.

These successful people will tell you 'I have done so much, worked so hard for my success.... And now I have everything that I could possibly want, *but* I'm not happy'. Or 'Something is missing, but I don't know what it is.'

To understand the wheeling and dealing that goes on inside the company 'I' somewhat better, we should examine the structure of the organisation more carefully.

The company basically has a top-down structure, so-called because it is almost completely directed from the top. But who or what is doing the directing? The direction is formed by the thinking and feeling mind, which can access two very complex instruments: the nerve system and a super high-tech chemical plant. These systems naturally interact, but the nerve system assumes the lead role.

The nerve system is unique. Any comparison does great injustice to life itself as well as to the greatest achievement of an undoubtedly divine nature.

Sometimes, however, one must simplify in order to understand. So we may imagine the nerve system as an enormous computer network linked by a very advanced telephone system.

This unique combination is designed to be able to perform at least 99% of its tasks completely unaided.

For instance, you never have to remember to make your heart or any of your other organs work, nor do you have to pay much attention to breathing or digesting your food, or to making waste products ready for excretion. You also automatically name almost everything that comes to your attention. Even when you are not working on a special problem , your mind is always filled with thoughts.

So this computer of ours is self-supporting and self-programming, as is the telephone system. When you accidentally touch something very hot, the telephone system initiates a very quick withdrawal for the hand from the dangerous place without any need for you to give it the slightest thought.

Let us stay with the computer for a while. With the computer we are dealing with programs and the way we can work with them. For illustration we will compare the nerve system with the computer.

THE 'ORGANISATION' MAN

COMPUTER	NERVE SYSTEM
We work with our mind on a computer and by doing so we make use of the available software	With our mind we actually work on our nerve system and here, too, we use the available software
Working on a computer we use software that we have programmed beforehand	While working with our nerve system we utilise what we have learned plus information the system has picked up on its own
Computer software may have bugs or viruses. In such a case the program will not run very well and the user will become frustrated at times; and will not get the required results.	In our nerve system all kinds of distortions may occur causing the mind to be unable to execute what it wants
The execution of tasks in a computer is managed by a built-in series of impulses. When other impulses get in or present impulses get out, the process changes completely. Sometimes, all of a sudden, a program loops its end to its beginning and the whole thing seems to run in circles.	Sometimes thoughts, too, seem to run in circles, returning every time to the same despairing point of view.

Here we will end the comparison between the computer and nerve system and concern ourselves with more interesting matters after, of course, having taken notice of the clear correspondences. Evidently the human brain that has created the computer is also a model for it.

An interesting question might be: Whatever can it be that influenced the programming of our brain in such a way that it often seems that life is filled with unsolvable problems?

What can it possibly be that causes some people to be almost always in a cheerful mood while others are often sad or depressed or seem to suffer from maddening fears or doubts about themselves. The answer in general is that this behaviour of the human brain was learned somewhere, some time in the past, and that this behaviour for the particular moment seemed the best solution for that moment's specific problem.

From educational psychology we know that the best and most intense learning takes places when as many of the senses as possible are taking part in the action: hearing, seeing, feeling tasting and smelling. A learning experience in which all these sensory impressions are active will dramatically facilitate the learning process.

When we talk about learning, there is no doubt that most people will think back to that particular activity we performed, or should have performed, at school, or during courses in which we participated. True learning, by which I mean severe, drastic learning, often takes place, however, under more stressful circumstances. Life's hard lessons are inevitably learned better and more decisively than those our teachers tried to make us learn. And this is because the lessons which life teaches us are usually spiced with *emotions*.

Our nerve system is an incredibly beautiful creation that has been built on several different levels. It developed along with our life form on earth. Deep in the centre of our brain lies a part that we could call our primitive brain, our limbic system. Medical science has not yet discovered very much about the way these areas work. The totality of the nerve system forms an exceptionally complicated system of very special cells.

At the deepest level of our primitive brain there seems to be a way of impulse-processing that is similar to that of the primitive animals. These primitive nerve processes are obviously still functioning in our full-blown human system, let us say, at the very bottom of our consciousness.

It seems true, or rather there is reason to believe that a part of our primitive brain, the hypocampus, forms the emotional centre of a human being. The hypocampus is a slightly cup-shaped part at the bottom of the brain. Underneath it, and connected with the inside of the cup, there is the pituitary gland. This is a small gland, not much bigger than a tiny grape, which we know plays a leading part in the endocrine system of the body. The endocrine system is the collective noun for all the glands in our body that administer hormones and similar chemical combinations to our blood. These hormones exert a strong influence about the way we feel. To summarise, we may say that both the hypocampus and the pituitary have a great deal to do with the way we feel.

In the past twenty years a good deal of medical research has focused on the workings of our nerve system and the way it interconnects with emotions. You may believe it or not, but very beautiful and interesting things have been discovered.

It has been known for quite some time that the nerve system, including our brain, consists of cells that can pass on messages to one another by moving small electric charges in a special way. Nerve cells can pass on impulses to each other, though not always. When they do, they can only do so in one direction.

The tiny spots where nerve cells can transmit impulses to others are called synapses. A synapse is a small space where one nerve cell comes very close to the next. To realise the one-way connection, the synapse requires certain protein-like combinations known under the collective heading of neurotransmitters and endorphins. Initially it was thought that only one combination, serotonin, was responsible for the connection. Later it was found that there were many more neuro-transmitters. It was also believed that these combinations only lived a kind of split-second life and that they disintegrated immediately after having made the connection. This is not completely untrue, because it happens very often, but not all the time and not everywhere. If it were to occur all the time throughout the nerve system, we would be forced to live like a new computer with no software at all. As you all know, a computer with no software is of no use to anyone.

Research carried out throughout the world has provided us with much new information. Whole series of neuro-transmitters and endorphins, as they are called, have been discovered. They seem to be produced in a way that depends on the *mood* of the moment in which one finds oneself. After reading about the hypocampus and the pituitary, you may have the same strong impression that I had as to the extensive interplay of these organs in producing these substances. More than sixty different neuro-transmitters have been found already, and it seems very possible and even likely that neuro-transmitters dedicate the path that nerve impulses follow in our body.

The funny and indeed remarkable thing about these phenomena is that everybody is familiar with the consequences of their existence. Let's just look at an everyday example.

John is a carpenter with a construction company. One day he walks across the building site with a heavy beam on his shoulder. Since he is talking to someone over his other shoulder, he fails to see the small hole in the ground into which, with his next step, he trips. A paralysing stab runs through his lower back. He can hardly walk, let alone work any more. The foreman sends him to the doctor, whose diagnosis is that John is suffering from acute lumbago. 'Tell your boss that you can't work for the rest of the week,' says the doctor.

'I'll prescribe you some muscle-relaxing painkillers. Come and see me again next week.' Because of the terrible pain, John has trouble getting home. In front of his house he sounds the horn long enough to make his wife, Rosie, come out and pull him from behind the wheel. John is in a very bad mood. To everything Rosie tries to say or do to comfort him he responds angrily and impatiently. Rosie goes off to do some shopping, leaving her grumbling husband to himself.

At seven thirty someone rings the doorbell. Rosie opens the door. It is Charlie, John's friend, whom he has worked with for years. Apart from being a skilful carpenter Charlie is John's best friend, and very gifted when it comes to telling the latest jokes. After having asked about John's back, Charlie tells one good joke after another. John roars with laughter. Every once in a while a shadow of pain crosses his face, but nothing worth mentioning. Without even thinking he gets up, as he always does when Charlie is around. He goes to the kitchen, gets two beer glasses, and from the bottom drawer of the fridge, takes out two cans of beer. He has to bend over quite a lot. He vaguely senses some stiffness in the lower part of his back, but he pays no attention to it. Armed with the two cans and the glasses, John returns to the living room. Charlie still has a few stories to make them laugh.

By ten thirty Charlie says: 'I'm off now. By the way, how's your back?'

'Well' says John, 'it doesn't feel bad at all right now'. The next morning at six, however, he can't get up. His back is giving him great pain again.

This story describes a series of events that everyone has probably experienced at some time. Something nasty has happened to you. You are in pain, in bed with a bad cold or flu and you feel dreadful. Suddenly something happens, a dear friend visits and your *mood* changes completely. Very soon you do not experience your pain and miseries any more. That is because the conscious part of our mind can only perceive seven plus-or-minus two items at a time. If and when the mood changes, new points of interest are chosen, while others elude our perception. They are barely felt or otherwise noticed.

Can it really be true that you only have to change your mood to get rid of a mountain of personal trouble? Yes, it really can! But . . . changing isn't all that difficult when you are dealing with an occasional passing mood; a mood you do not experience very often: let us say, a mood that arises from the uneasy circumstances of the moment, when of course such circumstances do not appear too frequently.

Soothing, for instance, is an action that is meant to change and improve the mood. It can substantially relax pain and tension. We see this very strikingly when, for instance, a young child has bumped his head and hurt himself. He cries in pain and self-pity. His mother takes him up in her arms and kisses the rising lump on his head and long before he is put down to play he has completely forgotten what has happened. The pain impulse has been disconnected by the gentle and pleasant perception of the soothing, thus altering his *mood*.

People are sometimes said to be inconsolable or heartbroken. Their whole being keeps on crying and mourning. The crying seems to be very important to them, for it goes on and on, profusely. In these cases, as the saying goes, bitter tears are wept. To understand the importance and the meaning of this process it is imperative that we pay attention to our faculties and needs to excrete. That is what the next chapter is about.

SUMMARY

Human functioning and perception are to a large degree directed by a system which uses small protein-like molecules, the neuro-transmitters and endorphins.

These substances are manufactured throughout the whole body, but mostly in the nerve-system itself.

With these substances, connections in the nerve system are switched on-and-off. These substances presumably also play an important catalytic role in and between the organs.

Neuro-transmitters are manufactured according to the mood or feeling which we are experiencing.

The field of our perception is limited: from a minimum of five to a maximum of nine items at one time. Our mood, good or bad, determines our perception.

Neuro-transmitters have a less limited life-span than was previously supposed. Insufficient 'healthy' excretion may easily lead to wide spread blockages in the nerve-system as well as in the rest of the body.

These blockages can and often do lead to mental and/or physical illness.

CHAPTER TWO

Excretion

All physical processes in which substance are transported out of the human body or to the surface of the body, for the purposes of removal, are called excretion processes. And since it is an incredibly well-organised company, we may be sure that these substances are removed for very good reasons. They consist, for the greater part, of materials for which the body no longer has a use and which would disturb the natural physiological processes if not removed. That is why the body transports them to places outside its own boundaries. There are also several substances which are really excretion products, but nevertheless play a more or less important role in the body's metabolism and other physical functions.

To make a company run smoothly it is important that there is as little contamination as possible. One might expect, therefore, that society would encourage these processes, that people would want to help each other to stay healthy.

In everyday life, however, we handle our excretion processes and products in a somewhat secretive way. It is therefore useful and enlightening to consider the excretion processes one by one and see what it means for our well-being if and when a process does not function optimally. It can also be instructive to find out how we experience each other's excretion processes.

Let us literally start at the bottom: the stool, the remnants after the digestion of our food, material we cannot use any more, together with, for instance, remains of old and therefore disassembled red blood cells, bile. At an average, civilised party the subject is hardly one for discussion. The popular expressions for these excreting actions are rather stigmatised and considered obscene. The use of these 'indecent' expressions will in almost any group cause disapproving looks. It is pretty much considered vulgar anyway to talk about this subject in polite society. Even more socially inadmissible are the consequences of, for instance, flatulence or wind. This can mean serious discomfort for a decent person who accidentally ate something she should not have.

The general attitude to the subject of fæces has led to a situation where, in every building in which one or more people need to stay for any length of time, private places called toilets have been installed, where a person can withdraw herself completely from the gaze and most certainly from the nose, of other people.

In places where this is not possible, people begin to retain their fæces. They enter a state of deprivation, as psychological science calls it, which means that they don't feel at ease or safe anymore. I know several people who for that reason never leave home for more than three or four days at a time, because they can't let go of their faeces anywhere but in their own home toilet.

Now, what does it mean for people's well being if they, whether consciously or not, retain their stool? In the first place, due to the growing mass, more and more water has to be drained out of it, to reduce the ever-growing volume. During this dehydrating process the fæces slowly turns as hard as rock, which causes the excretion process to be a painful adventure. Small pieces of this stony mass may remain in the lobes of the large intestine, causing severe contamination and malfunction and often even damage to the delicate mucous membranes. As a result of this all kinds of allergies may emerge, while the respiratory system and the skin can be heavily burdened due to the fact that they have to take over a part of the large intestine's job without being fit for such a task. Also dangerous are the chemical alterations in the substances secreted by the gall-bladder when they stay inside our body longer than 24 hours. Subsequently, if this is someone's normal condition, the natural motility of the intestine, which is responsible for the moving of the content, will slow down and even stop in the end. The large intestine is then completely paralysed. Any one who suffers from this can never produce a normal stool, but is forced to use laxatives all his or her life. Finally a longer than normal stay of the fæces in our body will cause the natural symbiotic intestinal bacteria population to shift towards a new and harmful population. Too often we see the development of fungi. The waste products that these organisms produce are in many cases pathogenic and even sometimes lethal to us.

In short, a badly functioning intestine spoils the joy of life and diminishes our life span.

The reason that we deal with our fæces so circumspectly may well be due to the fact that our primitive brain knows that our odour may give away our presence, thus making it easy for our natural enemies to track us down. Many animals bury their faeces for that reason. Doubtless you will now say that this danger for us in modern society is not relevant, which of course is true. But our ancient defence mechanisms and instinctive safety system do not let go so easily. Ever since we started living together under increasing crowded conditions, the urge for locks on toilet doors and sprays or air-conditioning for the elimination of odour has grown. We live so closely together that it is difficult to distinguish friend from foe. Instinctively we act in the 'better safe than sorry' way.

In conclusion it should be mentioned that in defecation we are dealing with a process which, at least in the beginning, can be influenced consciously, but which, when started, has a somewhat 'compulsive' element. It is hard to stop it before it is finished. Interrupting it feels very uncomfortable. This makes us feel vulnerable.

The passing of urine is to a considerable extent subject to the same feelings and restrictions. Due to the fact, however, that this process normally happens more easily and quickly, and because there is less odour involved, there are relatively fewer people who tend to withhold their urine. Quite apart from that it is virtually impossible to hold back urine for more than a day. Unlike the fæces situation, a person who feels the urge to urinate will do anything to create the chance, regardless of whom she's with or what he's doing, to release the stressing pressure in the lower abdomen.

If, for whatever reasons, the passing of urine is obstructed, a severe condition of toxicity will soon occur after which, if no adequate help is given, death will quickly follow. Urinating, too, is something we like to do in private, men a little less than women. Emptying the bladder, like defecating, is a process which really feels uncomfortable when interrupted.

The next excretion process is perspiration, sweating. The processes mentioned above have this in common, that we can control them more or less consciously. The degree of activity we undertake of course influences how much we sweat, but we certainly cannot control the process. Physical activity is a decisive factor, but the temperature of the air that surrounds us is also important, and we are not usually in a position to change that.

Sweat evaporates on the skin, which causes the skin to cool down. Transpiration gives us something like a boosted cooling system in cases where the body thermostat cannot handle the heat situation adequately. Furthermore the sweat contains important waste products.

How do we feel about people around us sweating? Well, lately it has become more accepted that it is a healthy habit to drive the foul liquids out of our pores every once in a while by exercising or going to the sauna. But there remains a considerable taboo on smelling sweaty. People who suffer from bad body odour are often avoided. The odour has to be masked by any means at any price, just like the other bodily odours discussed earlier.

It may be due to the fact that we cannot control sweating that the phenomenon is socially more accepted. We do not usually feel ashamed or stared at by others when we perspire. Sweating can partially but not sufficiently take over other excretion functions. When it is very hot, for instance, the production of sweat increases, whereas the production of urine diminishes. Also the composition of the fluid changes when this happens. Cosmetics to help the body smell better will not do any harm, unless the products chosen for this purpose are alien to the body, which, alas, does happen, due to the compulsion for manufacturers to come up with new scents every year. Consumers may be offered aggressive products which can impair skin function. The repression of the sweat function is very dangerous to our health. The total suppression of all sweat secretion is utterly dangerous. It deprives us of an important safety valve and may even cause death.

Incidentally, the odour that seems to come from perspiration is usually caused by gas-producing bacteria that live in and on the skin. The mere fact that these types of bacteria are so evidently present must be considered as a sign of a disturbed skin-culture. Since the skin tells the story of what's happening inside, bad smelling sweat should be considered as a general health problem rather than a phenomenon to be repressed on the skin. It should be remembered that suppressing any symptom whatever always makes things worse for you and in the end endangers your health.

Exhalation brings out gaseous waste-products. This is an excretion procedure which we can influence slightly, but which we cannot stop or interrupt. Cessation of breathing would normally lead to death within a few minutes. There is no social necessity to hide this particular form of excretion of waste products for the simple reason that the need to do so is inescapable. However, bad smelling breath is considered nasty and undesirable. Whenever this happens to us, for instance after having eaten a delicious meal richly spiced with garlic, we do almost anything to hide our breath, which alas we cannot. So we keep our distance from people and may even feel ashamed.

The excretion processes mentioned – defecating, urinating, sweating and breathing – all have, in a social sense, one thing in common. In all four cases we try to keep all signs of their occurrence out of the noses of others. It is considered totally undesirable that the odour of any of these processes should be smelled around us. We ourselves do not want to experience these odours from others. And when we do we label them unpleasant or even dirty. Odours make a strong impact on us and provoke feelings over which we have little control. All we can do is hold our noses when it is already too late. Other excretions that can sometimes be smelled and the sight of which alone may provoke responses like 'dirty' and 'inappropriate' are the mucus and wax excretions from lungs, nose and ears. We try to keep these excretions out of other people's perception. Coughed-up mucus is often swallowed or, like mucus from the nose, hidden away in a handkerchief. Ears are kept meticulously clean, sometimes so thoroughly that people damage their ear drums.

EXCRETION

We have two more products of the body which may be considered excretion products, but due to the fact that these products are so closely linked with our emotional state of mind, I'd like to speak about them in a separate chapter. They are saliva and tears. Before starting this treatise, however, and to stress the significance of these products, it is important to point out the ways in which our bodies' own excretion products can be used in a homeopathic way. This will be discussed in the next chapter.

SUMMARY

The fact that we try to hide ourselves during our excretion processes is only partially due to acquired behaviour. The instinct to hide everything that we excrete is an atavistic behaviour remnant from ancient history which was meant to conceal our presence from our enemies. That this is true is evident from the fact that we make a major effort to hide odour. Odours directly appeal to our feelings, our most ancient faculty. By constantly masking odour, or whatever comes out naturally, it is likely that we endanger our health and therefore the joy of life in a considerable way.

CONCLUSION

It might be desirable to be somewhat less inhibited towards excretion without, of course, letting go all accepted behaviour in normal society. To many people, a change in behaviour in a more relaxed direction would mean a considerable improvement to health.

CHAPTER THREE

Body's Own or Body-familiar Preparation Therapy

From several sources, especially the German natural healthcare literature, we are familiar with the use of the body's own substances such as blood and urine as a basis for the preparation of a 'made-to-measure' remedy. In order to understand this principle one needs to have some appreciation of the way in which homeopathic medicine works. This book is not intended as a study-course in homeopathy, so I will briefly explain how this gentle, curative method works, by using a few examples and describing some of the principles involved.

In orthodox medicine we are familiar with the fact that drugs often produce unwanted side-effects or, when the effect wears off, sometimes bring about a contrary-effect. To alleviate this the doctor usually prescribes a maintenance dose of the drug which has to be taken daily by the patient. This new dose is implemented as soon as the original dose no longer produces the desired results. Because of this, many patients, particularly psychiatric patients, continue the use of drugs for many years because they dare not risk the incalculable disaster that can occur when medication is suddenly discontinued. The same goes for sleeping pills. Cessation of sleeping medication after a long use will often cause the patient to lay in bed wide awake for a week or even longer: a very unpleasant outlook indeed. Thus large groups in our society depend on some kind of medicine and often more than one kind. If one considers people with chronic respiratory diseases, cardiac patients, people who suffer from rheumatism, and of course psychiatric patients, then we have a really large group of people depending on their medication. In many cases the prescribed drugs only suppress the symptoms of the disease. As soon as the patient interrupts the medication the symptoms return.

Followers of orthodox medicine may tell me now that the most important issue is that the patient does not suffer needlessly, and I agree with that, for those cases where there is no other possible solution. I think, however, that too often and too soon the search for real healing ends in daily medical routine and a real risk of drug dependency.

In homeopathic medicine the second or opposite effect of a medicinal substance is used. Toxic combinations, and we have many of them in nature as well as in chemistry, may have an ill effect on us when we ingest them into our biological system or often even when our skin is contaminated with them. Homeopathic medicine has discovered that toxic substances can often be used effectively in the preparation of very powerful non-toxic medicine. It is a known fact in non-homeopathic circles as well that toxicity diminishes and ends eventually by diluting the substance.

Avogadro, a nineteenth century Italian scientist, calculated that one part of an original combination, diluted 1:10 twenty-three times would not contain one single molecule of the original substance. The number 10 to the 23rd power is therefore called the number of Avogadro.

In preparing homeopathic remedies it is not unusual to dilute substances to an even higher degree. Opponents of homeopathic medicine find in this basic principle a reason to ridicule the whole method. More than once I've heard the sneer: 'Take a thimble-full of medicinal matter, pour it in a river, drive two hundred miles along the river to where it flows into the sea. There kneel down on the bank of the river and take out a thimble full of the water and here is your homeopathic remedy.' Absurd, they cry, the substance is long diluted into nothing. This cannot possibly work.

Concerning the degree of dilution, the opponents may have a point. A D2000 preparation has a degree dilution of 10 with 2000 zeros, which medical science considers to be ineffective. However the fact remains that homeopathic remedies actually work. For a better understanding of this you need to know in the first place that the high dilution degree in homeopathic medicine is not reached by diluting the original substance at once with a tremendous tank of water or alcohol. Dilutions are usually made step by step in 1:10 proportion. Every dilution forms the basis for the next. The diluting itself is done by a vigorous shaking of the fluid. The secret seems to be in the shaking. This shaking causes the dilution fluid, usually water or alcohol, to take over some of the properties of the original substance. While doing this, possible toxicity will eventually diminish. The truth of what so far might be called theory was proven by a simple scientific experiment, which I will describe. I have always regretted that the opponents of homeopathic medicine never bother to acquaint themselves with the outcome of this experiment.

The experiment was as follows. A concentrated dilution of a chemical water-soluble combination was made. A source of white light was used to shine through the fluid. A prism was placed which divided the light in the colours of the rainbow. This is called a spectrum. This spectrum was projected and a sharp image was made of it. In such a spectrum image some of the colours show dark lines. The substance in the solution absorbs certain wave lengths of the light shining through. The position of these absorbing lines is typical for every substance. So substances can be recognised by looking at their absorption spectrum. The resulting absorption lines in the spectrum are in such a case typical for what was dissolved in the fluid. What is held back in frequencies is like the handwriting of the substance.

Then, in a similar way, two more spectrum analyses were made: one from a normal solution with a diluting degree over the number of Avogadro, and here no typical absorption lines were observed; and a second one from a homeopathic dilution, in the same diluting degree as the one before, and well over Avogadro's number. This second dilution still showed some of the important absorption lines. This experiment proved the probability that in homeopathic preparation the essence of the original substance is transduced to the dilution liquid.

Spectrum analysis is very commonly employed by astronomers, where is used as a method to establish which elements are probably present on stars throughout the universe. They analyse the light properties.

So many 'magicians' pupils' like myself have tried to come up with a comprehensive scientific model to explain why and how homeopathic medicine works. There is, for instance, a German physician, Hans Heinrich Reckeweg, who states that a homeopathic remedy brings about a defence reaction in the organism against the remedy itself, and that this reaction, if the remedy is rightly chosen, resembles the defence reaction that is taking place in the body at that specific moment. But since there is no real need for defence against the harmless remedy, the sick person can have the profit of a doubly accelerated defence mechanism. This theory has been adapted by many workers in the homeopathic field. Well, I think there is much truth in it, but in an energetic model there is probably a little more to be said about this.

When I try to understand in what way a homeopathic remedy works in our body, I have to come up with a metaphorical example. When we are healthy, all kinds of, at first sight chaotic, electric patterns are observable throughout the whole body. It all appears very chaotic, but it isn't. When, for instance, we measure acupuncture points with a sensitive electronic device, as I did, we find very distinct values which only change when the person gets sick. In such cases we often observe something very peculiar happen. The skin resistance at the specific point we are measuring may increase while we are measuring it. And since this phenomenon is repeatable, it is clear that we are dealing with a valuable parameter.

When we place an ampoule of an appropriate remedy in the hand of the person we are measuring, and we measure again, we can observe the remarkable fact that the increasing skin resistance no longer occurs. What happens here should be considered to be one of the most wonderful opportunities to achieve a better understanding of the ingenious and very subtle working of the energetic beings that we are. Processes taking place in the sick body obviously show, as a measurable result, a lack of electrical balance. This balance can be restored by taking the right 'something' in the hand (or in the mouth). A 'healthy' body does not show any of these electrical imbalances. The restoring factor in the end can only be an electric or electro-magnetic one. This influence on the energetic balance is the special property of these homeopathic potencies. There is a huge number of restless oscillations in place, an electrostatic field, an absorption spectrum with a number of 'dark' places – the dips – in which the body can fill in its excess frequencies.

I realise that talking about frequencies and electrostatic fields belongs in the realm of physics. So to try and make these things more generally accessible I have come up with a story which I hope draws parallels.

Imagine a molecule of a noxious substance in your body. Now compare this molecule with a flock of sheep. To keep the flock together, the sheep dog has to run around it with a certain rhythm or frequency. Here the dog is the frequency that keeps the flock together.

Now let us imagine a homeopathic remedy. We'll compare that to a food which is very attractive to the dog. The dog finds the food and stops running around his flock. After a while the individual sheep will spread around, no longer under control. Since it was the flock as a unit which was the noxious molecule, you can easily understand that when the consistency disappears, the toxicity will too.

Now I would like to give a few illustrations of the way a homeopathic remedy works in daily practice.

If someone were to drink the juice or eat a few leaves of the foxglove (*digitalis*) his or her heart would start beating more and more slowly, while the volume of blood pumped with every beat would increase. (Orthodox medicine uses the chemical imitation of digitalis for people with a weak and irregular rhythm.) If this person took too much digitalis, death could occur because the heart would not be able to cope with such a strong stimulus.

In homeopathy, the preparations of this herb are used for just the opposite reason, that is an irregular or palpitating heart. In such cases the homeopathic dilution of the juice is often the right remedy. Compared to the expected effect of the juice, a poisonous substance, we observe that this drug has just the opposite property

Drinking the juice or eating the leaves of the blue monkshood (*aconitum napellus*) will soon make a person feel very restless. The skin will become hot and dry, the temperature will rise and heart will start beating faster and faster. The eyes may burn and limbs ache. In short, the person will develop flu-like symptoms.

Someone who is really getting the flu and showing the symptoms I have just mentioned will respond positively within a few hours to the administration of aconite.

Homeopathic medicine provides remedies made from substances which -in their toxic properties – resemble the existing symptoms. With homeopathic remedies one stimulates defence mechanisms that run strictly parallel to the mechanisms that are already at work in the patient and which provide reinforcement to the immune system of the body.

Apart from homeopathy which, as we have seen, uses very strongly diluted substances, we have the method known as isopathy. The word *homeo* means *resembling*. The word *iso* means *alike* or *equal*. In isopathy we use the same preparation techniques as in homeopathy. Here, however, the basic substances used are those which have already intoxicated the body. It is always possible that remnants of an intoxication or infectious illness were not completely excreted at the time the patient recovered. These remnants can and often do cause chronic health problems. So in isopathy we use not only toxic substances such as environmental pollutants that may have contaminated us in the past and that have probably accumulated in our bodies, but also bacteria, viruses and so on, especially in those cases where illness was treated with massive doses of antibiotics.

The healing effects that can be experienced from isopathic medicine, for instance the so-called nosode therapy, are often astoundingly positive.

When we use the body's own substances, such as blood or urine, as a basis for the preparation of a homeopathic remedy, we are working according to the rules of isopathy. Blood and urine may contain toxins which the body continuously fails to excrete.

Thorough experimentation has shown that excretion of these substances can be stimulated by giving the patient an isopathic preparation of his or her own blood or urine. As a result the toxic effects will diminish. Here we are dealing with a custom-made medicine*

---

*Whole libraries worth of material have been written about homeopathy and isopathy. I would encourage anyone who wants to learn more about these subjects to seek further information than can be provided by the limited objectives of this book.

SUMMARY

Homeopathy and the healing methods derived from it, such as isopathy and the body's own preparation therapy, work according to an energetic absorption principle.

There is nothing mysterious or exceptional about the way they work. Sciences like astronomy, physics and, in particular, modern electronics have, in contrast with medical science, been used to working with these principles for decades. These principles are also applicable to all living organisms. The remedies which are administered to a patient cause an energy field with useful 'empty' space. If and when the remedies are well chosen, noxious substances can be energetically neutralised. In this way they loosen their affinity with the body and can be excreted.

CHAPTER FOUR

Tears

Throughout history tears have held a special place amongst those substances we excrete. This may be because a flood of tears is so clearly related to our emotional state. Fairy tales and other stories of enchantment often contain accounts in which tears fulfil a magical role and sometimes even have magical properties

In the Bible there is a Psalm (56) in which tears are spoken about. The context in which the tears are mentioned here leads to the supposition that we are dealing with something of a profound nature about which I would like to speculate. Here is a quotation from Psalm 56, verses eight to ten:

> Enter my lament in thy book
> store every tear in thy flask
> Then my enemies will turn back
> on the day when I call upon thee:
> for this I know, that God is on my side,
> with God to help I will shout defiance.

A unique text, I hope you will agree. I suppose that many theologians will consider this as a metaphorical text, given that much of the Bible is indeed written in pictorial idiom. But let us, just for a moment, assume that we have a here a text with a literal meaning. What then would be the explanation?

In Israel (Palestine as it then was) the period in which these lines were written was a very turbulent and difficult one. As one can read in the Bible, the area suffered from continuing war and combat. The villages and settlements of the Israelites (then newly arrived) were under constant attack by the people who considered that they had a prior claim to the land and did not want these foreigners in their country, taking all the best plots. There were robbery, murder and rape on both sides; vengeance and counter-vengeance. All together the whole process lasted for several centuries before a comparatively peaceful society evolved. All this is recorded comprehensively in the Bible.

Now if I try to understand the part of the psalm I have quoted in a different way, I must think of these people returning from their work in the fields or on long journeys with their sheep, far away from home. On their return they all too often found their tents or houses burned, their possessions stolen and their wives and children raped, murdered or taken away to slavery. It was a brutal period. Put yourself for a moment in a situation like this and it is not too difficult to imagine the state of mind these people got into when they reached home. It must have been a combination of grief and rage; blind rage which demanded immediate revenge.

Since Jewish history is so meticulously documented it seems logical to assume the existence of an educated upper class. Even for those who do not believe in God, Jewish history shows remarkably intelligent planning and guidance.

I can imagine that intelligent people at that time intuitively understood that those in the grip of blind anger might develop a compulsive need to destroy, but that in that way their effectiveness and mutual co-ordination would be impaired. Reading and understanding the history of these peoples it seems likely that this culture possessed psychological knowledge.

One brilliant example is the story from the book of Judges about the battle to conquer Jericho, under the direction of Joshua. Joshua receives the order to march his men round the city seven times during daylight hours. He has to start at sunrise, march on through the day without stopping till sunset and then stop near a well. So these men had no chance to drink or rest all day long, which would have meant twelve long, burning hot hours. The Bible does not tell us, but I think that by the end of the day the weak men would long since have gone home. At sunset only the strong remained.

When we read on in the book of Judges about the battle of Jericho we see that the choice of the warriors for the assault on the walls was made basically according to the way the men satisfied their need for water at a well after that long and thirsty day's march. It was based on the character traits expressed by the way they took out the water, either scooping it up with their hands or recklessly sticking their whole head into it – surely a shrewd way to tell the reckless from the cautious!

Joshua needed only the reckless men for his assault.

Let us make another assumption: that someone discovered that at the site of a disaster you should, while walking around and comforting the people involved, catch a few tears from everyone. These tears – of rage, of deep grief and above all of powerlessness– you then mix and shake with water and then give a sip of the resulting brew to everyone who has to go into battle.

Just imagine!

In my own practice I have often had the opportunity to observe the fantastic effects on the mind and emotional state as I administer homeopathic potencies of patients' own tears. The pain of emotion is alleviated, sometimes even immediately.

Back to the psalm. If something like the gathering of tears is to be done in an organised way, you have to have a system of recording, as is mentioned in the psalm:

> Enter my lament in thy book
> store every tear in thy flask.

From my own experience with tear therapy I could imagine that some of the pain, and particularly the greater part of the blind rage, could be taken away by this therapy, leaving the men still highly combative but in a more disciplined and effective way.

I find it hard to escape the impression that this writer is very sure that he has the recipe for victory here.

I am well aware that this contemplation on part of Psalm 56, which is called 'Comfort to the Fugitive' is an unusual and personal one. I hope no reader will take offence at my interpretation. I intend no disrespect.

Like all the other substances that our body conducts to the outside, tears are an excretion product and just as in the cases of faeces and sweat, the production of tears serves more than one purpose. Our eyes need to be kept wet to prevent the sensitive sclera from dehydrating. Each time we blink our eyes, and we do so hundreds of times a day, we moisten and nourish the window through which we see the world. Without the moisture of our tears we would soon lose our vision. People with deficient tear production have to use an artificial moisturiser for their eyes several times a day.

There are circumstances, however, in which our tear glands produce much, much more liquid than our eyes need for moisturising. Part of the surplus is drained out through a little sieve-like bone between the cavity of the eye and nose. So we have to blow our noses. But sometimes it happens that this abundant production cannot be drained away through this channel, and tears run over the eyelids and down the cheeks.

When the cause of the tears is not a dry, cold wind or any pathological or anatomical deviation, we are dealing with a form of crying.

You can cry with laughter or sorrow, shame, anger or regret, but it is always the expression of an emotion.

We have said that crying is one of the excretion processes. As with the others, the amount of conscious control that can be exercised over it is limited; and we usually try to hide it from the prying eyes of others.

It is easy to find all sorts of theories that help to explain why we feel shy about our excretion processes, or the evidence of them detectable by sight or smell. There are the usual cultural and historical reasons; other people will say that it all comes from our educational background. Psychologists will probably point to a certain feeling of vulnerability and loss of control over our normal physical functions in cases where people feel observed. Of course it is very interesting to find why we are so anxious to try and hide these natural processes from others, knowing that we cannot possibly differ very much one from another.

The consequences of concealment can, however, become serious when hiding means suppressing. Speaking particularly of tears and crying, there are certain moods in which we would rather not be observed by other people. These include sorrow, regret, pain and anger, especially when it is powerless anger. We often strenuously suppress these emotions when we feel observed or deprived.

To illustrate how enormous and dramatic the consequences of this emotional suppression can be, I refer to what I wrote above about retaining other waste products and the problematic consequences of so doing.

It is of the greatest importance to appreciate that toxic excretion products which remain in the body must in time lead to irreparable damage and danger to the whole person.

When toxic waste products accumulate in the body, gradually a number of physical complaints will arise, due to the fact that the waste can only be stored in places not really designed for the purpose; once contaminated these areas can no longer fulfil their proper functions.

Thanks to neuro-physiological and biological research in the past years, we now know that tears also contain physiological waste products. Many neuro-transmitter substances are found in tears. Evidently crying fulfils an excretion function for the entire nervous system. Substances of which a surplus exists in the nerve system are excreted using lots of water. To clean up very large or sudden surpluses we use alternative methods. Imagine yourself frightened or nervous: you may experience an intensified urge to urinate or defecate; or you may start sweating.

The American writer and psychologist Robert M. Sapolsky attributes this phenomenon to an attempt by the body to reduce weight to a minimum when fleeing. This may be an important issue. These waste products, however, have never been properly investigated for neuro-transmitter substances, but since the whole nervous system uses them, we might expect to find them there as well.

Evidence for the assumption that the composition of tears is not always the same can be found in the expression: 'she (or he) felt the tears burning behind the eyes', an expression which may well be taken literally. We sometimes produce tears, especially under less pleasant circumstances, that really do cause our eyes to burn, and leave them looking red. Even before the tears appear we notice a change in feeling in our eyes. If there were no change in chemical composition we would feel the same burning and be stuck with the same red eyes whenever we laughed until we cried, which clearly is not the case.

In order to make progress in developing an idea one sometimes has to make an assumption or presupposition not based on hard accredited fact. For what I claim in this book, and which I will illustrate with some case histories, I make the following assumptions.

In the nerve system, as in the rest of the organism, waste or excretion products are stored in places which were neither designed nor intended for the purpose, when the natural excretion process (crying) is regularly suppressed. The outcome of this is unfavourable to the whole organism.

As a physiological process, crying can be compared with vomiting and diarrhoea. In these processes, during a very short period of time, relatively large amounts of composed material have to be eliminated from the body.

All the advice I give below for an effective therapy is based on this supposition. The similarity I perceive in crying, vomiting and diarrhoea really is not far fetched. In cases of vomiting and diarrhoea we often see rhythmic muscle spasms; and in intense crying we can observe the same type of spasm.

A German researcher, Lothar Göring, examined the correspondences between severe emotional experiences and a phenomenon which he had observed on accurate X-rays of the limbic system. He saw tiny white spots which, on closer examination, turned out to be little vesica filled with fluid. Göring called these vesica 'perifocal oedema' and attributed their origin to heavy, unassimilated emotions. Göring also compiled a complete cancer atlas, because he saw a correlation between the origin and the place of manifestation of the cancer on the one hand, and the type of emotion represented by the location of the perifocal oedema, on the other.

It would distract us a little too much from the subject in hand to go deeper into his research, but I can recommend his work as being thorough and reliable.

Neorobiologists have found neuro-transmitter substances in the tear liquid. The same substances are found in the blood as well as in the shafts between the nerve-cells and the surrounding glia-cells (the cells that nourish the nerve cells). Neuro-transmitters are also present in the synapses A synapse is the space where a nerve cell passes on impulses to the next one. This is the task for which it was designed. Synapses are supposed to disappear quickly after being used, but in many cases they do not, thus creating a situation in their region in which a nerve impulse constantly follows the same path. The consequence is the creation of a predictable reaction pattern. This is in fact what also happens during a learning process.

The neuro-transmitters are small protein-like molecules that allow us to make an almost infinite number of connections within our nerve system. The Dutch philosopher and writer Piet Vroon wrote in his book *Wolfsklem* that the number of possible connections which could be made by the nerve system probably outnumbered the water molecules present on earth. When you realise that just one cc of water contains millions and millions of these molecules, you'll probably feel as dazzled as I do when thinking about the divine miracle that was handed to us for free when we were born.

Severe grief or other strong and threatening emotions may lead to a situation in which in our consciousness only fixed paths are used. This is the case, for example, with people who have suffered so much disenchantment that they are no longer able to feel any trust or belief in similar situations again. Such people often suffer from blockages in various realms of life.

Apparently they are unable to make a new effort to solve the real problem. In their consciousness, the result of every new attempt is predictable: failure!

From the experience we have gathered in the past few decades from all kinds of psychotherapy, we know that deep and intense crying may often bring great relief from inner tension and physical complaints that correlate with it, thus bringing peace and calm.

Apart from the application of tears as a basic material for the preparation of a homeopathic remedy, something I do now, I have seen in my practice wonderful examples of the wholesome influence of deep and intense crying. I would like to include one of these examples in this chapter, because it illustrates the power and meaning of crying so well, and does not fit into the chapter of case histories, as it involves treatment.

Years ago a woman came to my practice, complaining of agonising headaches each weekend. A weekend headache is a relatively common inconvenience, which sometimes derives from the fact that the rhythm of people's lives tends to alter during non-work days. They may go to bed later, get up later, eat at different times. And of course alcohol is a well-known cause of some types of weekend headache.

I treated this woman with every method at my disposal. Since I am a chiropractor I checked every vertebra of her spine. It did not bring the slightest relief. I took out Kent's *Repertory of Homoeopathic Materia Medica* and worked out one remedy after another. No result.

But the woman kept making new appointments. It was as if she knew I would finally help her.

One day I investigated the family circumstances again. In the previous appointments she had always said that she was very happy with her husband and children. Now she told me that she had two children but that there should have been three. Eight years earlier her eldest child, a boy, had drowned.

I asked her to tell me precisely what had happened. She told me that the boy, who was four years old, had been playing on the lawn on front of the house. Nobody had seen what had happened. The child had fallen into a ditch which bordered the lawn and had not been discovered until the afternoon. The people who took the child out of the water placed the little body on the grass.

'I stood there watching,' she said. 'It was just like I had nothing to do with it.'

I asked her if she had not picked up the child.

'No,' she said, 'I couldn't.'

The funeral had not made any opening in her shield. She had the feeling that nothing that had happened had anything to do with her.

I told her that she had never said farewell to the child, that in a way she and the child had never really parted, that she had never surrendered the child, painful though that might be, to death. And all of this because she had not touched the dead child. She had not felt that her son was no longer there in that small, pale, lifeless body on the lawn.

She nodded in agreement. 'You might very well be right,' she said.

I suggested to her that it might help her if she went through that horrible Saturday afternoon again under hypnosis, and relived the most difficult time in her life, and also that it would be a very emotional experience. Yet she agreed.

It took two successive sessions to teach this woman to relax and yield to suggestions. In the third session she succeeded in getting back to that terrible Saturday afternoon. While she was in a mild hypnotic trance, I asked her if she saw the child lying on the lawn. She nodded. Then I asked her to go to the child and pick him up. I waited until she confirmed that she had.

Then I asked her to feel that the child was wet and cold and lifeless, and made her confirm that she had felt it. Then I asked her to kiss the child and say farewell.

The moment I asked that question, the woman started crying. She cried in a spasmodic, uncontrollable way for almost an hour, during which time I did nothing but encourage her to let it all go. Everything was wet from her tears. The, suddenly, the crying stopped and she became very calm.

About a month later she called me on the phone and told me her headaches had gone.

Looking back at this case I am almost sure that the woman must have known, during all those years of headaches, what was really bothering her, but that in a way she had refused to see the need to yield to her grief.

However, just as the large intestine, having stored waste products in unsuitable places for years and years, will not let go of all contamination in the first bout of diarrhoea, neither will the nerve system let go of all stored neuro-transmitters in the first major crying-fit. In this case, one hour of intense crying turned out to be enough for the woman, but this is not usually the case.

People also suffer on occasion because, to a greater or lesser extent, artificial blockages are inflicted on them. Nowadays, many depressed or otherwise mentally or emotionally hindered people are treated for years on end with drugs which obstruct or block all kinds of processes in the nerve system. Many complain about burning or dry sensations in the eyes. These sensations are side effects of the use of many of these drugs, and result from diminished tear liquid production. In my opinion this is the final ingredient for ultimate disaster:

less tear fluid means a diminished capacity to dissolve waste products.

So in all cases where one of the side effects of the drug is diminished tear production, I sincerely believe that these drugs should be removed and replaced by others which do not show this specific side effect.

To cleanse the nerve system deeply and thoroughly of hindering neuro-transmitter waste products is a very profitable use of isopathy. In an earlier chapter I gave some explanation of the principles of this method. I have applied this easy-to-learn therapy successfully in many cases and in so doing have gathered comprehensive experience of the wonderful effects of an isopathic tear dilution.

The consequences of tear therapy, as I have developed it, are often dramatically freeing. The preparation is simple and inexpensive.

In the next chapter I will describe the method fully so that, with this book as a manual, you, the reader, can learn to apply it yourself.

The method and the technical requirements are simple. I have never seen any harm or side effects resulting from these remedies. And there is certainly much to gain by using this method. It would be foolish to monopolise such a method, or to make it needlessly expensive.

SUMMARY

Crying should be considered as a normal excretion process. The process is intended to cleanse the nerve system of an excess of neuro-transmitters which no longer have a use.

If we consider the tear liquid that is produced during a crying fit as an excretion product, this liquid can serve as a basis for the preparation of an isopathic remedy. The usual effect of giving such a remedy is a freeing of blockages which the patient has experienced as a variety of primarily mental symptoms.

The effect is probably due to increased excretion of the excess neuro-transmitters in the nerve system as a result of the therapy.

CHAPTER 5

The Method

If the method described here were not so simple, many people would already have discovered it. We often overlook the easy things and seek out the difficult, attaching more value to complexity. The erroneous idea that difficult problems can only be solved by finding difficult solutions is a wide-spread concept.

First of all, I will tell you what materials you need for the preparation of the tear remedies. In the very first place you need tears, of course. The tears that are best suited to the purpose are fresh. The word fresh may sound a little odd here, but fresh usually means that the product has just been produced. The best tears, therefore, are those that have just been collected from the cheeks of a crying person. To be able to do that you need a certain skill. More important, however, is that you are calm and committed to what you are doing. Later in this chapter I will say more about the attitude of mind.

I recommend you buy some new 50cc bottles as used for homeopathic remedies, with a dropper and a screw-top. Pipette bottles will do, too, but in order to make this type of bottle suitable for our kind of preparation, the glass pipette tube should be easy to remove from the lid without causing the lid to leak. Any good pharmacist will probably have both kinds of bottle in stock, and they are inexpensive. Further, you will need a supply of physiological salt solution (0.9% water solution of salt). The concentration of the salt in this solution is approximately the same as in our tear-liquid. So we make the preparations by using the natural environment of the tears. This has considerable advantage when we later look at the possibilities for administering the remedy.

Of course, we can make the salt solution yourself by mixing 9g of salt in 1 litre of water. In order to have a constant good quality physiological salt solution at my disposal, I prefer to buy it from the pharmacist. It is not expensive and saves me the trouble of weighing the salt myself. If you buy your solution from the pharmacy, make sure it contains no additives, just the salt and pure water is what you need. These are the only materials required.

When you start collecting tears from a crying person, he or she may stop crying, wondering what you are trying to do. People like reasonable explanations and so it might be sensible to speak with the people to whom you plan to apply this and discuss the great advantages of the therapy with them long before you lead and help them into a state of mind in which they feel free to cry. It may even help if you give people some information on paper. At the end of this chapter you will find an example that you can adapt to suit your own needs.

Crying people tend often to rub their eyes with their hands or a handkerchief, or cover their faces with their hands. Obviously you do not want this to happen because it spoils your only chance of collecting your basic material. Experience has taught me that it is better to sit beside a person with whom I am working rather than taking a position facing the subject. Sitting beside my patient gives me the opportunity to gently put my arm over a shoulder, or touch a hand in a comforting way, providing my patient with a safe feeling. The patient will feel less observed this way and will therefore sooner let go of inhibition.

THE METHOD

Sometimes people need to talk about their emotional problems for quite a while on a practical level. Many people find it difficult to talk about their real problems and when they start to do this in a matter-of-fact way they will probably feel a little safer. For you, as the helper, there are a few important factors to consider. You should realise by now that the person you are helping should stop resisting and yield to the deeper feelings. Sometimes hypnosis can be an effective way to take away the feelings of insecurity and lower the defence against releasing the tears. In other cases I encourage people to write down a description of significant events, and especially what they thought and how they felt when they took place. People instinctively know which are the important painful memories, but whenever you ask them to talk about them spontaneously they seem not to remember. When, however, they start writing, I am constantly amazed at how memories seem to be as if tied to a string. And when you start writing, you start pulling that string.

When the 'homework' has been finished, I ask the person to read aloud what has been written. The voice is the sublime instrument for conveying the emotions. The distinctively individual sound of one's own voice is the vehicle with which we carry our emotions outside our physical boundaries. By reading out loud the things one writes about the painful episodes in life, emotions are triggered and tears will flow in emotional discharge.

Long before I had the idea for the isopathic tear therapy, I often recommended to people with emotional problems what I call the 'write and read aloud method'. People who are able to get their emotions down on paper often find this way of dealing with pain and grief advantageous. It is also a safe and convenient way to look take an objective view of yourself and your problems. The only thing you have to do is read aloud what you have written Stop when you begin to cry, do not hold back. As the crying stops, start reading again.

When you have finished reading, you should put what you have written away for a few days. Then read it aloud again in the same way. After a few readings you will notice that painful feelings gradually disappear. For the best results using this method, a paper should be read as many times as it takes for no feelings to be aroused, and no more. Having reached this state of mind it may sometimes even be helpful to destroy your writing in a kind of ritual way. You could tear it up or burn it, telling yourself that this painful piece of your reality is over and done with.

The fact that this simple method has worked so well for a lot of our people has made it clear to me that the voice is one of the most powerful instruments we have to bring out our emotions.

But to return to the subject of this chapter: as the tears flow I encourage my patient to go on. The words you choose and the attitude you adopt may differ from case to case. You will learn really fast if you have love and compassion for your fellow human. It is important that you succeed in creating an atmosphere of complete safety for your subject.

As I continue with the explanation I will assume that you have succeeded in gathering a few essential tears in an open bottle, catching them gently from your patient's cheeks. (Don't forget to remove the dropper before you start.) Technically it is not difficult to do, but realise that tears may run rather quickly down the cheeks. It is important that your movements around the patient are calm and delicate. An impression of haste may spoil the atmosphere.

When you catch tears you should remember that it is not the quantity but the quality that counts. Try quietly to catch as many tears as you can, but while doing so know that one single teardrop, cried in the right state of mind, provides you with all the material you need. I have made excellent, effective remedies from a single teardrop.

In spite of our good intentions and our care, some people will immediately stop crying when touched by another person. They don't like being touched, they may live in a somewhat distant way. Sometimes they are able to cry when left alone. You may be able to speak to them, but if you persist or come too close they may shout out 'leave me alone' or 'stay away from me'. These people should have the bottle or, even better, an empty eye-bath, in their own hand. This will allow them to catch their own tears without being distracted.

Many women use eye make-up, men often use after-shave. These products may mingle with the tears. My initial thought about this was that these extraneous substances might have a negative influence on the effectiveness of my tear remedy. However this turned out not to be the case. This isn't really surprising, because the diluting process involved here causes these substances to excrete too. So, if eye make-up or after-shave should contain substances that influence a person to his or her disadvantage, the isopathic diluting will simply diminish that influence. There is no need to worry that the efficacy of a tear remedy might be reduced by other substances contained in the fluid.

When you have the basic material you need (and one drop will suffice), just ad about 10cc of physiological salt solution. This is sufficient for shaking but it is not so much that your supply will diminish too quickly. If you make this kind of preparation often you will soon notice that pouring the salt solution from a big bottle into a small one with a narrow opening can be difficult. Again, at the pharmacy, I found a plastic laboratory siphon, which I filled with physiological salt solution. You have only to squeeze the plastic bottle to have easy control of the amount of fluid that comes out.

In most homeopathic and isopathic preparations the manual process is done by shaking the fluid vigorously at least forty times. For this purpose I use a stool with a folded towel on the top. With the little bottle in my fist I slam it 40 times on the top of the stool. The towel is meant to prevent me from hurting my hand. When done correctly you will hear and feel the liquid splash in the bottle.

Most companies involved in making homeopathic remedies use automatic equipment to do so. Sometimes the preparation demands that the shaking be repeated quite a number of times. Personally, I prefer preparation by hand. As well as being inexpensive, it emphasises the personal approach better than a machine can.

For the preparation of tear remedies I use a method which is known in homeopathy as the Korsakof method. In this technique, after each shaking procedure the bottle is emptied. The few drops of liquid remaining in the bottle form the basic material for the next step.

This preparation technique is known in homeopathic circles as being both inexpensive and very effective. As soon as you have obtained the required dilution, stop emptying the bottle and top it up instead with the salt solution. Now your remedy is ready for use..

It is advisable to label the bottle with date, K-potency and probable prescriptive data. If you are in professional practice you could add the specifications to the patent's file.

Now to a very important consideration: how do we find the right dilution of potency? My experienced colleagues will need no help. They will be familiar with a variety of diagnostic techniques, ranging from the specifications of classical homeopathy via electro or accu-diagnosis to kinesiology, the use of the pendulum and so on.

THE METHOD

For readers who have little or no experience of these techniques I would like to offer a few suggestions to help you choose the right potency. We have at our disposal two methods of looking at a question: intelligence and intuition, both functions of our mind. Both can be reliable, although we might decide that intuition (feeling), being connected with the ancient and survival-related part of the brain, the limbic system, is preferable, as it gives us a sense of what is good and safe for us.

Let's start with intelligence, if only because we are used to understanding what we are dealing with. Here we have the rules of classical homeopathy, which tell us to use low potencies (3,4,5,6,8,10,12) to treat new or acute cases, and higher potencies (30 and higher) to treat chronic cases. Put simply, the longer the history of the complaint, the higher the potency you choose. As you will appreciate, preparation of the higher potencies may demand a good deal of your time. I can assure you, though, that their use is often very rewarding.

In my practice I noticed, however, that most people need a K-4 or K-7 potency to begin with (K = Korsakof). In homeopathy the correctly chosen potency brings the best and quickest results. Other potencies of the same remedy will work too, but not as quickly or profoundly as the right choice would. Also, we see good results by mixing low, middle and high potencies. In these cases you don't empty the bottle completely, but you store and mix what you want to use in a separate bottle.

The testing technique derived from kinesiology is one that is nowadays applied by quite a few lay people. It is a method, quite possibly an art, that forms a real synthesis between knowledge and feeling. It is also known by the name of "Touch for Health'. Some excellent courses and workshops for learning these skills are available throughout the world. The test results are quite reliable. Skilful operators of this technique find it invaluable when choosing an appropriate potency. The same goes for Vegatest and Electro-acudiagnosis. These, however, are techniques only applicable by trained experts, whereas kinesiology is relatively easy to learn and can be used anywhere without any tools. Readers who are not experts need not despair, however. You may not a be a therapist, and you may have no intention of becoming one in the future. But if it is so simple to prepare a magisterial remedy out of someone's tears, you are interested in trying. Success can easily be accomplished in a simple way. You can depend on the reliability of this method and your skill will increase with frequent practice. You must first appreciate that it will not work if you doubt it. There is a statement about doubt in general made by the Dutch philosopher Saswitha: 'doubt is the origin of every disappointment.' This means: Do not recheck your first clear answer. This will only create confusion.

There is a theory about the human mind which says that human consciousness consists of a great number of fragment-personalities. Sometimes these fragments live harmoniously together but at other times they fight or quarrel. At such moments you are confronted with inner tension and conflict. Each part of our personality has its own special area of interest in life and conducts its own tasks. You might like to consider mind-relations which are of great importance to the total personality such as health, family work, money, hobbies, authority etc. Happily, we have the means to communicate in a respectful way with most of these fragments. We can enter into dialogues or even negotiations if we want to with these fragments, although we should never forget they are all part of what we call 'me'. Normally these negotiations go on undetected by the conscious mind. It is possible, however, to take part in these negotiations consciously. What I am referring to is a very special kind of inner dialogue.

The communications model I am about to describe is no fixed recipe. It is more an indication of how you might attempt to work with your fragment-personalities, to select the right potency.

Lean back in your chair and relax. Let your thoughts have their own way, but do not pay any particular attention to whatever comes into your mind. Try not to concentrate on anything in particular. Do this for about five minutes with your eyes closed. You will probably become more relaxed and that is exactly what is required.. When you are in a relaxed state of mind your feelings (remember: the very old and surviving part of the brain) take a stronger hold over your thoughts. Then ask yourself in a very friendly way, without actually speaking: may I ask something from that part in me that knows what potency to choose? Now this may sound incredible, but generally it works well. After asking the question, there are four possibilities which may all automatically come to mind. You might hear or see a 'yes'; you might here or see a 'no'; you might hear or see a specific number. It might even happen that you hear and see nothing at all. When you hear or see a number, you have your answer immediately and for the time being you should not ask yourself more questions. If you should see a 'yes', ask for the number. Accept in this case the first number that comes to your mind, because the fragments of your personality are just as unpredictable and playful as we are. They easily become annoyed and they do not like to repeat things any more than we do. If your answer is 'no', give it some time. Refusal does not mean that the correct answer is not there, you have probably just chosen the wrong moment. If you should hear or see nothing at all, trust to your inner possibilities and be patient.

There may be some delay between the moment that you are able to catch the tears and the moment you can start preparing the right potency. That is why I advise you in any case to prepare a K-1 potency. Protein molecules, like neuro-transmitters, tend to disintegrate. If you prepare a K-1 potency you slam the most vital information into a liquid with a better tenability than with fresh tears. So now you have a situation in which it does not matter too much whether some time elapses between the moment of collection and the moment of final preparation of the remedy. What is important is that you treat the immense source of information in your subconscious mind in the same kind and respectful way that you like to be treated yourself. You will be rewarded abundantly for your trouble.

You will no doubt appreciate that with this way of seeking knowledge and information, much more can be obtained, but that is not the issue here. What is at issue is the fact that you have the chance here to find out how many times you have to potentiate or dilute the tears you have in your bottle. In Holland we have a diagnostic instrument called a bio-tensor. It works in a similar way to the pendulum. The use of this instrument is not difficult. In fact you may find making and learning to use a bio-tensor greatly to your advantage. So I have decided to write the next chapter about this subject.

To recap:

Tears + physiological salt solution shaken or slammed 40 times = K(orsakof)1. Empty the bottle and again add physiological salt solution. Slam or shake a further 40 times and you have K2, and so on.

The method of administering the remedy also deserves some attention. It is usually advised that all homeopathic and isopathic remedies are taken in a clean mouth and kept for some time under the tongue. This goes for the tear-remedy, too. The sub-lingual mucous membrane is known for its permeability. We have yet another possibility, which lies even closer to the source of the tears. Since the remedies are fabricated with a natural and wholesome dissolving-fluid which normally has a very good and cleansing effect in the mucous membranes of the nose, we may achieve even better results from sniffing them. As we saw in an earlier chapter, the nose has many sensors for scents and is thus deeply connected with the limbic system. The sniffing of a tear remedy should therefore be considered to be a very useful method of administration.

Finally, I was introduced to a third effective way to administer a tear remedy by a patient, who dripped the remedy into his eye. When a sterile physiological salt solution is used for preparation, this is certainly a good idea.

Apart from the tears, which play a leading role in this area, we have a few more body-liquids in which neuro-transmitters cohering with some emotions may occur: saliva, sweat and blood. The expression 'blood, sweat and tears' to describe almost unbearable circumstances speaks for itself. But if you know anything about the functions of saliva you will probably object that it is produced to be swallowed. It fulfils a very important task in the digestion process. And you are right, of course. Yet I think that sometimes we swallow too much; that, for instance, we often swallow what would be better spat out. Some people 'swallow' so much that it becomes indigestible, it feels like a stone on the stomach. Eventually it can even cause them an ulcer. And if they continue swallowing too much it will go to the liver. These are all good reasons for the expression 'get it out of your system'. If only we could say that and really mean it a little more often.

Since we have some trouble in dealing freely with our excretion products, spitting is also considered vulgar, rude and indecent, a mark of the uncivilised. The one opportunity we have to spit is immediately after brushing our teeth Yet spitting may often, more adequately than any other action, express our anger and contempt, especially when powerlessness is involved. People even sometimes say that this or that 'left a bad taste in the mouth' when speaking of something that happened to them.

Saliva produced under these circumstances is a fine basic material for the preparation of yet another important remedy.

However, many people are hardly able to show any feeling at all, except perhaps for the universal, superficial, feigned exuberance that is today's mark of a so-called civilised society. In such cases we need to use some creativity to find a way to obtain the right basic materials.

When we sleep we don't exercise conscious control over the expression of our emotions. Many people's dreams include experiences that are both vivid and emotional. These dreams may cause us to cry out with grief; indeed such experiences constitute a considerable part of the importance of dreaming. It is well-known that people cry out in their sleep. In dreams we may cry not only from grief but also in anger or fear. All the important emotions go through our minds when we dream.

The residues of these nocturnal emotions are found when we awake. They are the dried, condensed waste matter we find in the corners of our eyes; and in the saliva, which may taste unpleasant when we first awake.

It really is not very difficult to take the waste-material from the inner corners of the eyes and some morning saliva, and add a physiological salt solution. Left for an hour or so in this liquid, the grains from the eye corners will soften again, and with a little shaking their contents will dissolve into the liquid, thus providing the essential material for our remedy.

The saliva that is in our mouth when we awake is a very interesting material for preparation as well. I have seen good results in the resolution of old anger, using preparations from morning saliva.

As you can see, the preparation of tears or other isopathic remedies can hardly be called difficult. Whether you work with patients in a medical practice or do it just for yourself or the people around you, this simple technique will provide you with the means greatly to improve your mental and physical freedom and hence your physical well-being.

SUMMARY

To prepare a tear remedy

1. Catch someone's tears (maybe your own) in an open 50cc bottle.
2. Add just enough physiological salt solution to enable you to shake them.
3. Shake or slam the bottle vigorously at least 40 times.
4. Determine by your own most reliable method what potency you need.
5. Prepare the K. potencies by slamming each potency at least 40 times in the same bottle, pouring out every slammed potency except the one you need.
6. Top up the bottle with physiological salt solution and your remedy is ready for use.
7. Administer the remedy under the tongue and keep it there for a few minutes before swallowing, or sniff it up the nose.

A Short Explanation of Tear Therapy
(a page to copy)

Every part and function of our body creates waste-products while working. We have to get rid of waste in order to be able to function in a normal, healthy way.

Experiments have shown an increased rate of waste excretion if a homeopathic dilution of a natural waste product of the body is administered.

Tears contain superfluous waste products of the nerve system, their constitution depending on the mood in which they are cried. The presence of an excess of waste products in your brain and peripheral nervous system may easily leave you with blockages and inhibitions where there should be none. This might well have a negative influence on your spiritual and physical health.

There are good reasons for believing that the increased excretion activity generated by homeopathic dilutions as described may also be expected from tear dilutions.

Do not be shocked or surprised if the person you turn to for help catches your tears and prepares a wonderful remedy for you. If the opportunity is there, release your tears, as long as it feels good to do so.

If you need further explanation, just ask.

CHAPTER SIX

Diagnosis Using the Bio-tensor

This chapter contains directions for the manufacture and use of a diagnostic device, the bio-tensor. The possible applications of this simple device will amaze you once you have acquired the basic skills.

Before writing about the bio-tensor method, I must state that it is neither more nor less reliable than kinesiology. With the latter method, however, it usually takes two people to get a result. The bio-tensor method of diagnosis can easily be applied by just one person. It is a good idea to find out which method suits you best.

This is another practical chapter, containing a good deal of information that you can apply in your search for answers to important questions. However, please read the whole chapter through first, before trying it for yourself or doing the exercises.

In Chapter Five I discussed some possible ways to find the right potency of a tear or saliva preparation. Writing this chapter I realise that, for most people, making an initial diagnosis is not part of their usual daily routine. It is a skill to be learned, not a trick which produces new and amazing results.

In this chapter I want to introduce an instrument that will help you make a diagnosis. In my view most people can readily learn how to use it. You do not need special skills to make this tool yourself.

In Holland, where live, the bio-tensor has been on the market for several years. It should be considered an extension and improvement to the pendulum, which is in fact no more than a wire or a thin chain with a small spherical weight 'pending' from it.

Figure 1 shows a pendulum and a bio-tensor. The price for a skilfully manufactured bio-tensor varies, but may be quite high. However, I hope to show you that you can produce an excellent instrument yourself with a few bits and pieces which you can find around the house.

But before showing you how to do this I will explain how and why it works, give you an insight into the purpose of the bio-tensor and show why the exercises I describe below are necessary.

The bio-tensor, like the pendulum, is no more than an extension of your hand. Both instruments are made to magnify, and so make more visible, the small, involuntary movements of the hand. The name consists of two parts: *bio*, the first syllable of the word biological, and *tensor*, which is derived from the verb to extend. A *bio-tensor* is thus something designed to extend the possibilities for recognising numerous biological processes, in short: diagnosis.

With training one may even be able to use the bio-tensor to find answers to questions in the psychological or spiritual area, which is possible if we manage to make the connection with our subconscious inner source.

In using the bio-tensor, and of course the pendulum, it is often assumed that the human organism works like a very sensitive antenna which registers every signal, no matter how low the intensity. Furthermore it is assumed that every signal has its influence on the whole of our organism and thus on our involuntary patterns of movement. The patterns of movement, or more precisely, the changes in patterns of movement

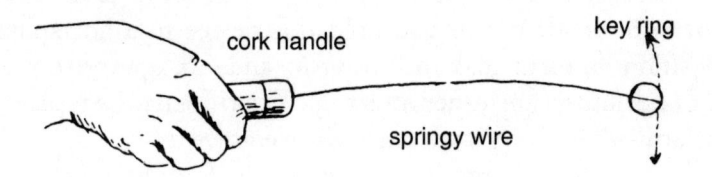

DIAGNOSIS USING BIO-TENSOR

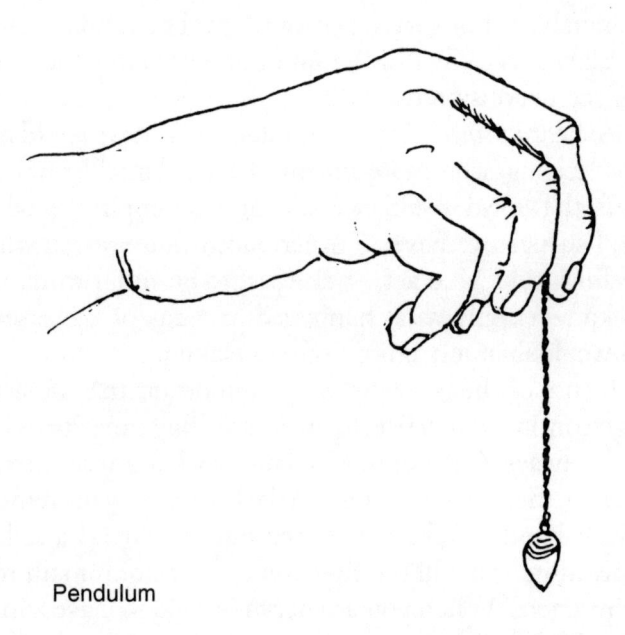

Bio-tensor — cork handle, springy wire, key ring

Pendulum

Figure 1

meant here are so insignificant, minuscule, that they are not easy to detect.

As you can see in the picture, the bio-tensor consists of a handle with a springy wire. On the other end of the wire is metal ring. The weight of this ring is chosen so as to make the wire bend. When you hold this device in a horizontal position you can make it swing to-and-fro, up-and-down, around, and in any other direction. The ring may be replaced by any other object with the right weight.

In an earlier chapter I wrote that one of our most important sources of knowledge is our ability to feel. Feeling, in all its complexity, is one of the main activities of our limbic system, the system which has provided organised life on earth with a reliable set of survival parameters. The limbic system, which allows us to feel, is the safest and certainly the oldest part of the nerve system.

I once heard a wise friend of mine say that if we could only trust our feelings a bit more and our so-called intelligent brain a bit less, the world would be a safer and better place in which to live. I suspect we have all experienced situations in which our feelings told us to act, or else just to be still. I think that we all know exactly what happened in many of the cases in which we deliberately ignored these feelings.

In the use of the bio-tensor, it is important that we learn, through continued practice, to link our feeling capacity (which is nearly always right) to our involuntary hand movements.

You may think that you don't make involuntary movements with your hands. Well, just stretch out your hand and look carefully at it. You will see that you cannot hold it still for a single moment. When you are nervous, i.e. you have a lot of uncontrolled feelings, the movement of your hand will be even stronger.

The exercises described here are meant to link those in-

DIAGNOSIS USING BIO-TENSOR

voluntary movements to a significant set of meanings. If we train with careful consistency, our bio-tensor will develop into a useful and reliable aid.

But before we can train and practise, we need to acquire a bio-tensor. A simple version will do just as well as the most expensive one. For this simple device you need the following materials:

1. Three or four wine bottle corks
2. Approximately 50 cm springy wire
3. A solid key ring
4. A few drops of quick-drying glue
5. A small piece of sandpaper

Instructions

Insert the wire lengthways through the corks, keeping the corks to one end of the wire.

Apply one two drops of glue between each cork and press the corks together. Make sure the wire does not protrude from the last cork.

You can now sand the corks until you have a nice handle, from which about 40cm of wire extends.

Slip the key ring onto the other end of the wire so that the wire goes between the two circles of the key ring. When you pick up the wire by the handle the wire will bend. Now you can make it swing. By sliding the trapped key ring up and down the wire you can find a swing speed that feels right in you hand.

Why must it feel right? The answer is that I would very much like you to have a bio-tensor that you enjoy using. It should become a device that you like to hold in your hand

and play around with. From experience, I know that the swinging speed of a bio-tensor is a very important factor as to how it feels and whether you are inclined to work with it or not.

When you have found the right position for the key ring, cut off the length of wire that protrudes beyond the key ring and fix the ring with a few drops of glue. Now your bio-tensor is ready for your first exercise.

Exercise 1

Hold the bio-tensor in a horizontal position with the ring straight, as shown in *Figure 1*. The arm should not be completely stretched, but slightly bent and held forward in a relaxed way.

Make the ring swing up and down only, and try to control the movement. Make sure the swing keeps going with the same amplitude. As soon as you are able to make the bio-tensor swing in the exactly the same way for at least half a minute, you may proceed to the next exercise.

Exercise 2

The instructions for this exercise are almost the same as for the last, except for the direction of the swing. Here you make the bio-tensor swing from side to side. When you have succeeded in making a consistent swing for at least half a minute, you may go on to the next exercise. A word of advice: be really critical with yourself. These exercises won't work if you take them lightly.

When you have acquired sufficient skill in the first two exercises, your bio-tensor can already 'say' two words. Maybe you will decide to call them 'yes' and 'no', though it may be a little too early for such a decision, as you will see.

DIAGNOSIS USING BIO-TENSOR

Exercise 3

This is a comprehensive exercise and I advise you to practise for ten minutes a day for at least six weeks. The more dedication you put into your exercise, the more reliable your work with the bio-tensor will be.

Hold the bio-tensor in your normal, relaxed starting position, which is horizontal, and look at the ring. Now *imagine* that the ring will swing up and down. Don't move your hand, just think. After a few seconds you will probably see that the bio-tensor gradually starts swinging in the direction that you want, although you are not aware of any hand movement.

When you have succeeded in achieving this, try to get the same result in other directions. In fact you should try, just by looking and visualising, to make the bio-tensor change to any movement that you hold in your mind.

When you succeed in this exercise you will notice that the bio-tensor 'listens' better every day, until you reach the point of total control, which is the moment when your bio-tensor quickly produces any movement you think of.

The moment has now arrived for you to find out when your bio-tensor means 'yes', when it means 'no' and when it means 'maybe' or – which is very important – 'I can't help you with this question'. To find the yes-and-no swing you need to say something that is absolutely, verifiably true or not true, so that you can calibrate.

Take the bio-tensor in your hand and hold it in the normal start position. Then say: 'I am (now state the name of another person)'. Now you have said something that is absolutely untrue. Look very carefully at the movement your bio-tensor makes at this very moment, because this movement means 'no'.

Repeat the action, but this time state your real name. Watch the movement by which your bio-tensor says 'yes'.

You have now reached an important phase in your bio-tensor training. You have made the first big step in linking your bio-tensor to the vast resources of your subconscious mind, which includes the entire realm of feeling

The only remaining task left is to learn to trust yourself completely in what you are doing. Faith is not so much something you have to earn; rather it is one of the most important pieces of equipment in your inner tool box, which undoubtedly makes the chemistry work.

Doubt, on the contrary, is the one and only emotion that can and will bring about failure and disappointment. Never ask the same question twice while working with your bio-tensor. If you do, your subconscious mind will conclude that the first answer was wrong, because it has no sense of so-called scientific experimentation. Its nature is simple, plain and honest. Repeating questions will create confusion, which is a state of mind that will gradually undermine your training.

Exercise 4: Linking to other people

This exercise has to be done with the help of a second person. First you have to find what I call the 'I' point. You may remember a situation in which you were accused of something, or maybe something was said about you that surprised you, and you said, 'Who? . . . me?' at the same time tapping your sternum with your index or middle finger. This sternum point I call the 'I' point. I find it best to touch this specific point on the person's sternum with the fingers of my free hand in order to establish the contact I need for work with the bio-tensor. In the other hand is the bio-tensor at the start position. To be able to ask questions about the other person, the only thing you have to do is keep in touch with the 'I' point and wait for the bio-tensor to say 'yes' This attuning procedure is imperative if you want to make a useful diagnosis. If need be you can also do this exercise on your own. It can be useful in establishing a clearer contact with your own inner self.

It is not essential to use your writing hand to work with the bio-tensor. I have know people who were definite right-handers, but had to use their left hand to get satisfying results when using the bio-tensor. You have to find that out for yourself. I advise you not to debate this with yourself, just *feel*.

The selection of potency with the bio-tensor.

Before we can select the right potency, we have to find out whether the basic material, the tears in our case, is worth working with. If the basic material is not right or not as good as it should be, we may be heading for disappointing results. The tears we gather have to contain sufficient neuro-transmitter substance of the type that should be washed out of the system. To check our basic material, we can use the bio-tensor.

A well known fact in bio-tensor technique, as well as in kinesiology, is that our system can provide us with both 'in' and 'out' information. This means that we are able to find out if a substance corresponds to a toxic or unhealthy substance inside the system. The part of the body on which to rely for information on any substance needing removal from the organism is the area above the collarbone, except for the ears. So if you want to find out whether the tears you have gathered in your little bottle are the right material for the preparation of a homeopathic dilution, place the bottle in the person's hand and ask them to hold it against their forehead, which means that your basic material is in touch with that person above the collarbone. Look at your bio-tensor and when it says 'yes' you have the 'right' tears, ones which are worth potentiating. When, however, the answer is 'no', it is better to wait for another opportunity to gather useful tears.

When you have the right material, have the person hold the bottle against the stomach. In our questioning system this means: 'Do you want the material in this form?' To this question the bio-tensor should say 'no'. Having arrived at this stage of your diagnosis you can choose to opt for a slow or a quick procedure. The slow procedure is to test the potencies one by one, holding them to the stomach. When you are well-trained in this work it is sufficient just to mention the potencies while the other person holds the bottle to the stomach and you keep contact with the 'I' point. Although this is a quick procedure it is imperative to wait a few seconds after mentioning the potency. For example, you say: 'K1', wait a few seconds; the bio-tensor keeps saying 'no'. You say: 'K2', the bio-tensor still says 'no', and so on, until the moment the bio-tensor says 'yes'. Then you know which potency you have to prepare.

As you can understand, the touching of the other person's 'I' point at the start of the procedure and the waiting for the 'yes' links your subconscious mind to that of the other person in such a way that you can act as your patient's diagnostic instrument.

After having read all this you may decide to *buy* a bio-tensor. There is no real argument against such an intention. Beautiful instruments are available. The disadvantage is that they are more expensive. I personally prefer my own self-made and balanced bio-tensor to the commercially made products that I sometimes see a colleague using.

Working with the bio-tensor can be a revealing and rewarding experience.

CHAPTER SEVEN

A Few Case Histories

I can't very often claim that the people I have treated in a particular manner or at a particular time have all reacted positively to my therapy. The cases described here represent a more or less random selection.

Due to the way in which I keep notes on the reactions of my patients to the different types of therapy I apply, I can easily evaluate the therapeutic results of my work. As a professional therapist I find it important and also rewarding to keep a critical eye on my own work.

We all like to refer to our successes, but complete or partial failures are less pleasant, though equally important, to admit. Failures are important because they provide the best opportunities for learning.

It is also a good habit to discuss the ups and downs of one's work with one's colleagues, even those who seem themselves to have nothing but successes. They, too, may have something to add to your own methods and opinions.

When it comes to the tear therapy I can declare honestly, and to my own amazement, that I have not had a single negative, nor indeed zero, reaction. Undoubtedly the tear therapy, like every other method, has its limitations. I just haven't been able to find them yet. So I hope you will understand and excuse my enthusiasm.

TEARS

First Case History

A woman of about thirty came to my practice for treatment. Her story, as is the case with most of the people I see, begins with a description of her physical complaints. She is constantly tired, her muscles ache, she seems unable to concentrate on the work in hand. She has had to give up her job in a clothes shop because, as she puts it, she cannot walk about, even for half an hour, 'I feel really sick, dead tired', she says. 'Everything hurts.'

I write it all down and ask her questions. She tells me that she has lost a lot of weight over the last few years. In the good times she used to weigh 116 pounds. Now it is only 94 pounds.

Only a year ago I would have had my diagnosis ready at this point: this looks very much like M.E. (myalgic encephalopathy), also called post-viral syndrome, a commonly occurring disease today with few possibilities for treatment using orthodox medicine. Undoubtedly her physical symptoms pointed towards this problem. Now, however, I would like to have a bit more of her emotional history.

So I enquire about her childhood and in particular her schooldays. She tells me that she had a terrible time at school. It all started in kindergarten, when she was four. She had a severe squint in one eye and was pestered badly because of this. She didn't feel supported. No-one ever stood up for her. When she was a little girl her mother was always ill and needed every bit of available attention for herself.

While we are talking, I ask her to *be* that cross-eyed girl in the kindergarten again. With this woman no special communication technique is needed to take her back to the past. It seems as if all the wounds in her mind are still open and that she has waited all these years to let go of her tears. She starts crying desperately, like a child. Carefully I put my arm round her shoulder and tell her that what is happening is good.

I encourage her to let go of all her negative emotions, aware of course, of the neuro-physiological impossibility of her doing so, because a single emotion will always take the lead in the ongoing process. The encouragement is simply designed to take away any possible remaining inhibitions.

While my patient continues to cry, I carefully take one tear after another from her cheeks with my open bottle. I test her kinesiologically and find weaknesses in all family relationships, which means that negative stressing factors characterise her family ties.

She tells me that she was treated for two years by an electro-acupuncturist, and mentions his name. I know the man: he is one of the best there is. She also tells me that his treatment resulted in the excretion of lots of toxic waste from her body and my very skilful colleague told her that he was very sorry but that he could not help her any further.

Subsequently she had been treated by another valued colleague, who used Bach flower remedies. These normally beautiful remedies had affected her adversely and she had got worse again, which is a rare phenomenon.

'You are the last straw I can clutch at,' she cried to me.

Now you may think that we have here a lady with a certain talent for drama. And of course you are entitled to your opinion.

However I have learned that while some people's behaviour may look like play-acting, there is actually a good deal of truth in amongst the posturing. In cases of real posturing there are so many inconsistencies in the behaviour, which will be evident to a trained observer. When we are faced with consistent behaviour, play-acting is less likely.

TEARS

The woman didn't look well: her face was reddish and puffed-up. The electro-acu-diagnosis I made showed very high values overall, which usually means that every function measured has great difficulty in keeping up with the needs of the system.

I prepared and tested her tear remedy and subsequently administered a few drops under the tongue. Then I asked her to go back in her mind to that miserable kindergarten experience and stand again in the middle of the circle of name-calling teasers.

'Can you see and hear yourself there?' I asked her.

'Yes, I'm right in the middle of it,' she said.

'Please tell me what you feel.'

'Well,' she said, 'you may think it strange, but actually I feel nothing at all.'

In other sessions I have noticed this striking effect: the almost immediate disappearance of all negative sensation from the totality of a memory, once the tear remedy has been administered.

A few days later the woman called and told me that something strange had happened almost immediately after she took the drops. She said: 'I was sitting on my sofa and took the drops. Within five minutes I fell asleep. I slept like a log for a good hour and woke up soaked with sweat. Is this a normal reaction to this therapy?'

I explained to her that the heavy sweating was probably triggered by an enhanced excretion reaction in her body and that sweat is a very useful carrier in ridding the system of waste.

These symptoms of sudden sweating and sudden sleep stopped after about a week. Later the patient visited me to have a tear remedy prepared from 'other levels', as she called them. On these occasions she brought her own, self-prepared K1 potency, since I had taught her how to do this.

Now, four months after we started the therapy, her vitality has increased remarkably. She looks much better, having gained 14 pounds, and is thinking of taking a job again. Of course she still has problems to solve, but her attitude to life is more balanced and she feels she can manage on her own now.

Second Case History

Another very remarkable case was that of a young mother in her late twenties. In the past I had successfully helped her to get rid of her spinal complaints. Now she had a completely different kind of problem. She was worn out, due to a total lack of sleep. Her oldest child, a boy of three, kept crying night after night, coming to her bedside and waking her up several times in the course of a single night.

The family doctor had examined the child and had found nothing disturbing or requiring treatment. 'And now,' the mother told me, 'I can't help myself. I am simply beginning to hate my child.'

It took just a slight gesture of compassion from me to bring out her tears. For this reason it seemed very useful to prepare a tear remedy for her.

After I had prepared and tested the remedy I explained to her that it might be a very good idea to make such a remedy for the child too. I told her how to gather his tears, which was unlikely to be too difficult since he was there, crying at her bedside several times a night, and how to prepare a K(orsakof) 1 potency. Such a preparation is more viable than pure tears. Neuro-transmitters are a kind of protein and tend to decompose outside the body, whereas the K1 already has the most important information shaken into the salt solution.

So I gave her a clean bottle and a 10cc ampoule of physiological salt solution. We agree that she would return on the day she was able to collect the tears from the boy in her little bottle. I also asked her to bring an object that the child cherished and kept by him, at least at night.

Many children have a Charlie Brown-like security blanket, or a special soft toy to which they are especially attached. In kinesiology such an object can be used as a diagnostic tuner.

A few days later she phoned and I asked her over the same day. She brought the K-1 of her son's tears and his 'security blanket'. She told me that she already felt much more at ease after having taken her own tear remedy.

Using the objects she had brought I made a tear remedy for the child. Now this may seem a little unusual, but in kinesiology we can make a person a test subject for someone else. To do this we need any object that is more or less constantly in the proximity of the person for whom we are doing the test. In this case the security blanket worked just fine. So, for the duration of the test the mother became the child. In this way I succeeded in making a suitable tear remedy for the little boy.

I advised the woman to administer ten drops of the remedy to the child every day and add just one of her own drops to his remedy. In homeopathy we have the 'rule of mother and child'. The bond between a mother and her child is such a strong one that we often see much better therapeutic results when we treat both, in cases where one of them is ill.;

A few days later the mother phoned me again. She told me that something wonderful had happened, which was illustrative of the mother-and-child rule.

'He slept much better with his drops,' she reported, 'but when I added one drop from my bottle to his, he slept the whole night through and was very well behaved during the day, too. I think this is fantastic,' she concluded.

A few months later we met again and she told me that she had mixed the drops exactly as I had told her. 'There is a new closeness between him and me that I have never felt before,' she told me.

This mother discovered that after this therapy the relationship between herself and her child was strengthened and improved. From everything I have seen in this respect I have to say that my work never ceases to amaze me and make me feel grateful for such a beautiful and lasting result.

Third case history

Sometimes people's lives are completely ruled by their family or their in-laws. This happened to the young mother in this case history. Her own mother had died from cancer; her father suffered from cardiac disease and the only attention he paid was to his own problem; her husband was a workaholic and her parents-in-law were so domineering and preoccupied with themselves that neither of them would pay attention to anything she had to say. She felt completely isolated and imprisoned.

Apart from specific symptoms she complained about being so very tired.

'You know what I really hate about myself?' she said. 'I clean my house over and over again to make sure everything is tidy, but with my children I can't seem to do anything but snap. I act very impatiently towards them, which I don't want to do. I wish I could hug them and play with them in a cosy way, but I can't and I don't know why.'

This situation had grown so out-of-hand that this woman seemed unable to be her normal emotional self within the family. All the family did to her was demand, without any rewarding warmth, appreciation or even attention.

It was not difficult to let her cry, as she was desperate, tired and humiliated..

Once again I had the opportunity to prepare a suitable tear remedy.

A few weeks later she reported that her attitude towards her children had greatly improved; the atmosphere was much better. She was able to act much more independently towards her in-laws and was no longer so affected by their lack of normal attention. Her pathetic father no longer had a hold over her. Physically, she still suffers from some symptoms, but her chronic fatigue has eased.

Fourth case history

I achieved quite an interesting reaction from a physician. A week earlier I had given a lecture to a group of physicians who work with bio-resonance techniques for diagnosis and treatment. It was a pleasant and very perceptive group of people. I lectured to this group about the tear therapy and the simplicity of preparation of the remedies.

Everybody in front of me industriously wrote down what I said.

A week later, I met the same people at a seminar given by a well-known German colleague. One of the doctors, a woman of about forty-five, told me that during a crying fit she had caught her tears in a paper handkerchief. She had placed the handkerchief on the input antenna of her bio resonance device. On the output antenna she had placed a small bottle of water. She had used this water as a remedy. 'After taking these drops, I dreamt for the very first time in my life that my mother was kind to me,' she said.

CASE HISTORIES

For me this was a truly striking example of the impact of this therapy.

I could present more case histories, but I think what I have written so far is actually sufficiently illustrative. I trust, however, that the above mentioned stories may encourage the reader to apply this therapy and subsequently produce his or her own case histories.

Think, for instance, what magnificent help you can offer little children who cry easily whenever they panic. Among many other situations, panic is often seen in little children when they are taken to hospital. Fear can be such a torture for these little ones.

We can think of so many situations in which people find themselves in agony or grief for a period of time, during which they often cry. The mourning period after the death of someone we love is a very good example of such a situation. The help you can offer is of great value, but will cost you hardly anything more than the compassion you already feel.

CHAPTER EIGHT

Conclusion

As you have seen, maybe from your own experiments, tear therapy and saliva therapy are not difficult to master. I cannot conceive of any insurmountable obstacles to the successful application of this therapy.

I have to say, however, that no single therapy, or healing method known today, is a cure-all panacea. Yet I am sure that this method contains important elements to help bridge the gap between mind and matter.

I hope you have understood the importance of your attitude at the moments when you gather tears. The composition of tears varies with the mood or state of mind a person is in. When we try to help someone by making a tear remedy, we must avoid altering this person's state of mind. In other words, we must try to suppress our natural tendency to soothe and comfort the crying person. Instead, it is better to encourage the crying and to try to support the other person's present state of mind. This way there will be a strong excretion of the neuro-transmitters linked to the state of mind, which provides us with excellent basic material.

It may sound dramatic, but it is recommended that you encourage people to really yield to their misery. The more deeply they let themselves go, the more suitable your basic material, the tears, will be in the preparation of a powerful remedy.

In the chapter about the method, I described a case of a

mother whose child drowned. In the period directly after the child's death, the mother withdrew herself from emotional involvement. She had not really cried, thus inhibiting the excretion of abundant neuro-transmitters. This woman suffered for years from severe headaches, starting every Saturday, the day she lost her child.

In this last chapter I would like to put further emphasis on the importance of crying when it is needed. The case that I am about to describe, like the case of the mother, was one I encountered before I discovered the tear therapy.

This case history is about a middle-aged man. He came to see me about his increasing headaches. For several months he'd been unable to do his job as a controller in a large company in Utrecht.

As in the case of the mother, I felt I was groping in the dark as to the cause of his disease. And just as I did with the mother, I started to treat him according to my normal standard procedure.

Quite soon his condition became aggravated. He almost lost the courage to go on. He said: 'I know that I won't get well; it is hopeless, and I don't believe anybody can help me'. This, of course, pressed me to a more thorough inquiry.

You may wonder whether it is my habit to examine the state-of-mind of my patients in a superficial way. Well, it is not, but in our profession we have to be very prudent. In my part of the world people tend to hide mental problems. When they are ill, they like to be simply, understandably and physically ill, in a way which enables them to say to their relatives 'I have this or that', meaning 'It has nothing to do with the real me; it just happens *to* me'.

So at the start I often have to gain the trust of my patients by doing nothing but treat physical problems in a physical way. Quite often that's enough. When a health problem is solved without having to talk about the chemistry 'between the ears' (as we say here, meaning it is all inside your head), people are greatly relieved. And when the simple approach works, it is not wise to go any deeper. People do not appreciate that.

In this particular case three visits had already passed and I had not progressed any further. I asked the man if anything serious had happened in his life in the last few years. He answered by asking whether it is was all right for his wife to come in from the waiting room. I told him that of course it was all right, but only if he really wanted her to come.

While he sat there in his chair, arms folded across his chest and head bent, his wife told the story. It was a sad one. The couple once had three children, a son and two daughters. The son, the eldest child, had been especially loved by the whole family. From the way his mother told the story it was obvious that he had been a reliable, hard working, but also a sensitive and loving person. He had always been ready to help anyone who needed his skills. He really was the joy and pride of his parents.

One Saturday evening he went out with his friends. They carefully made the deal about who was going to drive back home. As it was his turn to drive that evening he abstained totally from alcohol.

In the middle of the night they drove home. The atmosphere was relaxed. The three boys who had had quite a few beers felt really safe with their sober driver. Unfortunately, the driver of a big truck coming from the left had not seen the car with the four boys in it. The driver in the left front seat, my patient's son, was killed instantly.

The patient's wife, who told the story, said: 'My husband has never been able to accept the death of our son'.

The father had meticulously arranged everything concerning the funeral. He had written a long speech, which he had read at the funeral mass. Together with many of his son's friends he had organised the death watch for his son's body. During this whole period he had been strong, 'incomprehensibly strong' his wife said.

After the funeral the parents went to the cemetery once a week to take fresh flowers and tidy the grave. The father thought it only natural that his daughters accompany them, every week. But after three months the girls started looking for excuses to skip this weekly trip. The father could not understand this lovelessness and demanded that they kept coming, thus causing stress in his family. During this period his headaches began.

This particular father was unable to let go of his departed son and could not understand that his wife and daughters could.

I asked the man to write about the whole period of the death and the funeral, with special emphasis on what he had thought and felt.

The next week he came, bringing twelve hand-written pages. His wife sat next to him and he started reading.

He had produced an almost minute-by-minute report. Everything he had done, everyone who had visited, and what they had said. Every external move was in this report. But, he had not written a single word about his feelings. He read all twelve pages calmly and with a certain pride about how well he had done what had to be done.

I knew, almost from the moment he started reading, that this was not what I wanted from him. This was just the account of how a decent father had organised his son's funeral. Perfection in everything was very important to this man.

When he had finished reading I told him that he had done tremendously well, and asked him if he still had his funeral

CONCLUSION

speech in his possession, and if he could bring it for me next time.

The following week they came in and sat down. From the inside pocket of his jacket he handed me a bundle of paper. 'Here is the speech you asked for,' he said. 'You may read it if you want to'. I looked at the first page and saw that this was the right material. 'Well,' I said to him, 'I think this is about the feelings you really had at that time. I want you to read it.' He gave me a fearful glance. 'Do I have to?' he asked. 'Yes, I think you should,' I said.

During the funeral period his sense of duty had enabled him to push away his feelings, and had made it possible for him to read this very moving farewell speech for his son. But now, broken by grief, and upset by the reluctance of his daughters to visit the grave, which had deprived him of the certainty that he was doing right, his resistance broke down. He had hardly read half a page before, finally, the tears came.

Three more times the couple came back to have him read the speech. Every time he cried, but every time it was less grave than the time before.

Three days after his last appointment his wife called me and told me that her husband felt better and that he had accepted the attitude of his daughters. She also thanked me for my trouble and patience.

As you can see, again, the method of writing and reading can also lead to the healing of pain. With this man I succeeded in bringing him to a point of deep emotional excretion. However, to get the right results with this method, you need not only love, but a lot of time, skill and trust as well. For many people this is, although it works, too much and too heavy.

When we apply the tear therapy as described in this book, we also need at least one real emotional crying fit, to collect the right basic material. After this, however, the resolution of the problems usually goes more smoothly and more quickly. Good therapeutic results are easier to obtain. And please don't forget what was written in this respect about the morning saliva and the material from the corners of the eyes.

Sometimes it is advisable to begin the therapy using just these materials. It gives you a chance for a non-confrontational and non-threatening start, especially with people who have covered up deep inside them all the miseries of the past.

In our modern society we have developed the habit of minding just our own business, rather than other peoples. This is not entirely wrong when it is intended to live and let live in mutual love and understanding. Meddlesomeness and nosiness are generally not valued. But in too many cases, the fear of these qualifications has turned people towards carelessness and lovelessness. It is all too often 'every person for him or herself' nowadays. Through this social development we seem to have forgotten that we are not meant to be alone.. We need each other, which means that every human being has to do quite a bit more than just minding his own business.

We are creatures with a very long history. The basis of our thinking and doing is – and has always been – our mood, or state of mind, what we feel. We are interdependent, we need each other badly. Therefore I invite everybody who has read this book to give its contents and meaning a warm place in their life. Don't hesitate whenever you really can be of help. Just act as you know how .

Can you imagine how glorious it feels when someone says to you: 'I feel wonderful and happy, and I am finally me. Thank you for helping me.'? I can assure you that it is one of the most marvellous things that can happen to you.